GW00467682

Oregano Oil

Nature's Answer
to Bacterial, Viral,
and Fungal Infection

Candace Salima

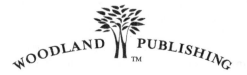

WOODLAND PUBLISHING
™

For order information or other inquiries, please contact us:
Woodland Publishing
448 East 800 North
Orem, Utah
84097
Visit us at our Web site: www.woodlandpublishing.com
or call us toll free: (800) 777-2665

The information in this book is for educational purposes only and is not recommended as a means of diagnosing or treating an illness. All matters concerning physical and mental health should be supervised by a health practitioner knowledgeable in treating that particular condition. Neither the publisher nor the author directly or indirectly dispenses medical advice, nor do they prescribe any remedies or assume any responsibility for those who choose to treat themselves.

ISBN 978-1-58054-475-7
Printed in the United States of America

Contents

Contents

The Story of Oregano

Oregano is in the Labiatea family, (mint) and closely related to basil and marjoram.[1] It takes approximately 200 pounds of oregano to produce 2 pounds of oil of oregano. Now, you might be asking yourself: "Oregano? Isn't that in my spice cabinet? Don't I use that in my pizza sauce, spaghetti sauce, or to flavor a multitude of culinary delights?" Yes, you do. But, as with almost every spice or herb used in cooking, it also has many wonderful healing properties.

The oregano commonly used to spice up meals is not really oregano, but generally marjoram, thyme, or Mexican sage. The real oregano has a powerfully overwhelming smell and a slightly bitter taste. When fresh, the flavor is so intense it will leave the tip of the tongue numb. Marjoram is sweeter and is often the spice used for pizza sauces and the like. So increasing your intake of what you think is oregano just won't produce the desired results.

However, medicinal oregano oil has been proven to assist in the eradication of a number of pesky health issues that plague many people. In this booklet we will thoroughly examine oregano and its key constituents to understand better its many uses and applications.

Oil of oregano is derived from the wild oregano species (*Origanum vulgare*), a plant that is native to the mountainous regions surrounding the Mediterranean, especially Greece and Turkey where it has been used for centuries. The three strains of oregano proven to hold all the necessary healing properties are lumped together and called P73. Oregano also must be emulsified in a carrier oil such as extra virgin olive oil, coconut oil, or one of equal integrity. Several studies have demonstrated a wide variety of beneficial uses of oil of oregano which support claims long purported by folk medicine practitioners.

Oil of oregano has a lot of uses. It functions as an antibiotic, anti-fungal, antibacterial, antiviral phytonutrient and is also a powerful antiseptic used both internally and externally. Specifically, oregano oil has proven antimicrobial activity against food-borne pathogens such as *Listeria monocytogenes*.

To benefit from the key active constituents of oregano—namely, naturally occurring antioxidants, phenolic acids and flavonoids—make sure you're taking the genuine article, not just another spice with the same name! Real oregano is rich in calcium, magnesium, zinc, iron, potassium, copper, boron, manganese, vitamin C, vitamin A (beta-carotene) and niacin, just to name a few nutrients.

Because of its broad range of uses in health issues, we'll look at oregano from both the perspectives of modern medicine as well as folk medicine.

So, make yourself a warm cup of chamomile tea, curl up on the couch, and let's learn a little about this common seasoning found in nearly everyone's spice cabinet.

Modern Medicine and Oil of Oregano

Many medical practitioners are finding that the oil of oregano is use-ful in the fight against bacterial, fungal or viral diseases. The key ingre-dients in oregano oil are carvacrol and thymol. Both carvacrol and thymol are phenols which have been credited with having antifungal and worm-expellant properties. These powerful phenols compose 90 percent of the constituents of oregano oil.

Oregano effectively kills bacteria, fungus and viruses as well as par-asites. This natural germ fighter may even offer some hope in combat-ting the growing problem of antibiotic-resistant bacteria. Science has been studying both oil of oregano and crushed oregano for decades. One challenge is that there are thirty to forty species of oregano, which leads to the confusion in finding those that actually do have healing properties. Most do not. The effective strain—medicinal grade oregano—arises from a specific species that grows wild throughout the world. The highest grade, or rather, the one with the strongest con-centrations of carvacrol, grows wild in the Mediterranean region.

To find genuine oregano "with healing in its wings," carefully research the provider's ingredient source. Only the strain that grows wild and is identified as true oregano has been extensively studied and only it has been proven to produce the promised benefits.

"All species of true oregano belong to the mint family. However, there are dozens of species plus a variety of subspecies. Of the sixty-plus species of oregano or oregano-like plants, relatively few possess significant medicinal powers," writes Dr. Cass Ingram, author of *The Cure is in the Cupboard*.

It is a very powerful oil and should not be ingested or applied to the skin unless the following criteria have been met:

- Be certain it is derived from a Mediterranean species (P73 wild oregano). Medicinal oregano or wild oregano is rich in essential oils, rare and difficult to procure.
- Be certain it has been tested and its thymol levels are low. (There are numerous species of oregano that have higher levels of thymol and are, therefore, toxic.)
- Be certain it has been tested and proven to have high levels of carvacrol, the major healing element in medicinal oregano.
- Be certain it has been tested and is confirmed pure and free of adulterants.
- Be certain it is diluted in a carrier oil, such as olive or coconut oil.

Most oil of oregano produced in the United States is actually marjoram or thyme and relatively useless. So, make sure the oil you use is indeed distilled from the P73 blend, a true oregano.

Conditions Aided by Oil of Oregano

Conditions that have been proven to be helped via numerous scientific and medical studies are as follows:

Acne: Hormones, diet, microbes . . . there is still speculation about what causes acne, although a host of possibilities are readily available, such as unbalanced hormones—the bane of teenagers and menopausal women. In most cases, the sebaceous glands—the tiny oil glands found on the face, neck and upper chest—become overactive and then are infected by various microbes (usually staphylococcus bacteria).

Whatever the cause, oil of oregano has had an enormously wonderful effect on acne. A tiny drop of oil on a pimple—morning and night—will cause it to quickly disappear. A drop or two of oil added to your cleanser will do as well. However, oil of oregano has a natural drying effect and that is a problem for women with menopausal skin. So experiment carefully and see how it works for you personally.

Animal/Venomous/Insect Bites: Any bite from a dog or cat, spider or reptile (snake etc.) can quickly become infected, causing serious illness. As soon as possible,wash the wound thoroughly and when necessary, seek medical attention. Saturate the bite with oil of oregano and repeat the application several times daily. It not only keeps infection from developing but can also help stop the bleeding.

Asthma: Asthma is a chronic condition that occurs when the main air passages of your lungs, the bronchial tubes, become inflamed. The muscles of the bronchial wall tighten and produce excess mucus, which causes the airways to narrow. The incidence of asthma has reached epidemic proportions in the United States.

Nearly five hundred thousand Americans with asthma are hospitalized every year and thousands more die. Although doctors claim the cause of asthma is unknown, it has been traced to allergens. Severe allergic reactions to a multitude of foods, dyes, sulfates, MSG, artificial colors, and processed vegetable oils. Oil of oregano, with its anti-inflammatory, cough suppressing, and healing properties, goes a long way in easing the suffering caused by asthma. Try rubbing the oil on your chest or inhaling the vapor directly from the bottle.

Bed Sores: Anyone who lies incapacitated for any length of time will suffer from bed sores. This is why nurses turn patients often and why physical therapy is so important. Not only are they trying to keep muscles from atrophying, but they are attempting to keep circulation flowing throughout the body. People with diabetes or poor circulation are also likely to suffer from ulcerations of the skin. Once a person has a bed sore or ulceration, there is greater risk for infection. Oil of oregano fights infection in open wounds as well as stimulates quick healing. Apply the oil directly to the wound and cover it with a sterile bandage.

Bronchitis: Bronchitis occurs when the inner walls that line the major air passageways become inflamed. While modern science merely shrugs its shoulders and says bronchitis follows a cold, other sources place the blame for bronchitis strictly on molds. Antibiotics kill only the bacteria, which is a minor cause of the inflammation, but unless they kill mold and fungi, too, the bronchitis will continue. Oil of oregano will kill any bacteria, mold, or fungi residing within your bronchial airways. To kill mold in the air, add a few drops to hot water and spray the room. To kill mold in your bronchial passage, inhale the vapor directly, or take an oregano supplement internally.

Burns: Oil of oregano is potent when treating burns. Its anti-inflammatory powers quickly relieve swelling and pain. There may be pain in the beginning, because oregano is a hot oil, but dramatic improvement will result from its application. Applied directly to the burn, the oil halts blistering and sterilizes the burn so it can remain free of infection while it heals.

Canker Sores: Canker sores are a sign of a malfunctioning immune system. They occur primarily in the mouth. The most likely source of canker sores, according to some doctors, is a bacterium, group A strep. Applied directly to the sore, oil of oregano—as well as L-lysine—has proven its ability to kill group A strep.

Cavities: Cavities are holes in the teeth caused by plaque, a sticky substance made from mucus, food particles and bacteria. Brushing and flossing remove plaque and are critical to good dental health. Oil of oregano, because of its powerful antibacterial action, fights plaque and helps prevent cavities.

Coated tongue: The tongue is a breeding ground for harmful bacteria that attack not only your teeth, but your tongue as well. Oral thrush, now known as oral candidiasis, is the main culprit of a coated tongue. It produces a bad smell and a white coating on the tongue. In adults, it is a sign of a severely depressed immune system and you should see your primary care physician for a thorough physical. Babies contract it because they may have a weak immune system. Taken internally and used in a salt water gargle, oil of oregano easily kills this infection.

Cold Sores: These sore and painful lesions are caused by herpes, the same strain that causes chicken pox. Stress, infectious illness, food allergies, alcohol abuse, drug abuse, and a host of other sources trigger cold sores. While oil of oregano has been proven to kill this virus without pause, L-lysine also is quite effective against cold sores. The oil is extremely strong, so don't apply more than one drop to the sore.

Common Cold or Flu: Every year, tens of thousands of people suffer from colds or flu. It seems to be a yearly plague that hits us about late fall and generally lasts through spring. It's annoying, uncomfortable, and sometimes embarrassing. Colds and flu are caused by infection. Taken internally, oil of oregano is a powerful antiviral agent.

Cradle Cap: Cradle cap is crusty, scaly skin on a baby's scalp. According to the Mayo Clinic, it is often due to seborrheic dermatitis. It generally appears in the first twelve weeks following birth and rarely continues after age one. A drop of oil of oregano in shampoo will helps rectify the situation.

Crohn's Disease: Crohn's disease causes inflammation in the small intestine. The inflammation extends deep into the lining of the affected organ causing constant pain and diarrhea. While no one really knows what causes Crohn's disease, the prevailing theory holds that the body's immune system is reacting to a bacterium or virus. If this theory holds true, oil of oregano taken internally could be an answer to the problem.

Croup: Croup is a respiratory infection that causes the larynx or trachea to swell due to infection. Once the larynx goes into spasms, the individual will have difficulty breathing, experience a harsh, barking cough, hoarseness, tightness of the lungs, and feelings of suffocation. The essential oils in oregano have a cough-suppressing effect. In addition, the infection will be eradicated with oil of oregano's antiviral actions.

Dandruff: Most people don't know this, but dandruff is actually a fungal infection. Fungal infections and scalp conditions like this are often partially a result of some kind of deficiency. It doesn't hurt to begin taking supplements such as fatty acids, B vitamins, biotin, riboflavin, or zinc. This can often take care of the deficiency, especially with a few drops of oregano oil in a dollup of shampoo. This one two punch can often knock the fungus out cold.

Diarrhea: Diarrhea can mean many things because it is a symptom of numerous disorders. Both parasitic and bacterial infections can be blamed for diarrhea. Some of the few microbes that cause diarrhea include salmonella, shigella, camphylobacter, clostridium, giardia cyclospora, tapeworms, pinworm, flukes, cholera, *E. coli*, enterobacter, flu virus, *Candida albicans*, cryptosporidium, amoebas, hookworm, and roundworm. Again, the microbe killing power of oil of oregano is phenomenal and has been proven not only in numerous studies, but the U.S. government has also found it extremely useful in killing microbes in septic water. Take several drops of oregano in water or juice a few times a day for the best results.

Diverticulitis: Nearly half of Americans over the age of sixty have bulging pouches (diverticula) in their digestive tracks. If you have these pouches, you have diverticulosis. Diverticula usually form in the intestines. These, in and of themselves, do not usually cause problems. If diverticula become inflamed or infected you have a condition called diverticulitis. This condition causes severe abdominal pain, fever, pain, nausea and causes marked change in your bowel habits. Because the cause of this condition is infection, whether bacterial or viral, oil of oregano can kill the infection and ease or eradicate the symptoms. Diverticulosis will remain—diverticulitis should not.

Ear infections: While it is true the ear can be infected with fungi and bacteria, a common source of ear infections is food allergies. If you have reoccurring ear infections, go to an allergist and be tested to find your specific allergies. In addition, if the source of the ear infection is fungi or bacteria, again, oil of oregano taken internally can kill the source and clear up the problem.

Eczema: Eczema is skin disorder resulting in itchy inflammation and rashes. It has long been regarded as an allergic disorder. Cow's milk is a common cause of eczema in babies. Researchers have discovered that a deficiency of fatty acids and vitamins are a common factor in eczema sufferers. But even more so, researchers at the University of Tennessee discovered that eczematous lesions are infected with several varieties of fungi as well as staph and strep. In their study, they discovered once the fungi, staph, and strep were killed, the eczema cleared up.

Erysipelas/Cellulitis: Erysipelas is an inflammatory disease of the upper layers of the skin. Cellulitis is an inflammatory disease of the skin and deep underlying tissues. Group A strep germs generally cause both diseases, and oil of oregano has been scientifically proven to kill strep.

Symptoms of cellulitis may include fever, chills, and swollen "glands" or lymph nodes. The skin is painful, red, tender and may blister and then scab over. You may also have perianal (around the anus) cellulitis and may cause itching and painful bowel movements.

With erysipelas, a fiery red rash with raised borders may occur on your face, arms, or legs. Your skin will be hot, red, and have sharply defined raised areas. The infection may come back, causing chronic swelling of your arms or legs (lymphedema). Applied directly to the skin, oil of oregano can kill the microbes causing the cellulitis. However, a physician should always be consulted when cellulitis is contracted in order to get immediate help in the form of an antibiotic because this disease can lead to blood poisoning, even death!

Folliculitis: Folliculitis is infection of the hair follicles, which appear as pimples or non-healing crusty sores. An acute eruption for a short period of time is usually due to a staph infection and can easily be treated with oil of oregano applied directly to the affected area. Extended reactions generally take place where shaving, waxing, hair plucking, or friction occurs. If folliculitis appears, it is best to cease these actions immediately and allow the hair to grow in naturally before resuming. If necessary, an experimental treatment of laser hair removal provides an alternative that relieves the skin in the long run.

Frostbite/Frostburn: Extended exposure to cold temperature will result in frostburn (chilblains) and then on to frostbite, a painful and serious condition that sometimes results in the loss of toes and fingers. Oil of oregano is a hot oil, and like cayenne, which should be administered internally when hypothermia sets in, oil of oregano can be put directly on the frostburn or frostbite. It can increase circulation and will dramatically improve the circulation, thereby minimizing tissue damage, as well as reducing inflammation and relieving pain.

Furunculosis/Boils: Furunculosis is a condition causing deep sores of the skin, also known as boils. Boils are an infection of the skin. Boil come in two kinds: furuncles (infection of the hair ducts) and carbuncles (infection of the sebaceous glands). Both are caused by bacteria infection with staph being the most common source, although strep o *Candida albicans* could also be the root of the problem. Apply oil o oregano directly on the boils to get them under control.

Gastritis: Gastritis, the inflammation of the stomach lining ma cause a gnawing or burning pain in your stomach or upper abdomen This can be caused if you take excessive amounts of aspirin or othe pain relievers that irritate your stomach lining. Drinking excess amounts of alcohol can also cause this. However, studies have shown that gastritis can also be caused by the same microbe that causes stomach ulcers, *Helicobacter pylori*. Gastritis is often a precursor to stomach ulcers, so take care of the gastritis immediately and save yourself the pain and trouble of dealing with the ulcers. Oil of oregano will kill *Helicobacter pylori*.

Headache: The use of oregano as a treatment for headaches goes back centuries. Inhalation or rubbing of the essential oil on the temple and over the sinuses is a quick reliever of headaches. Headaches have a variety of causes, though allergies are often the culprit. Even migraines can be traced to an allergy of some kind: molds, foods, environment. Find the source of the allergy and the headaches often go away. Until then, keep your oil of oregano handy.

Head lice: These annoying bugs have a special taste for humans. Head lice general result from poor hygiene or exposure to someone with head lice. The antiparasitic properties of oil of oregano quickly dispatch head lice. A few drops of oregano oil added to a small amount of your shampoo should do the job. You can also add a few drops of oil to your wash cycle to take care of any lice that find their way onto your clothes.

Hepatitis: Hepatitis is inflammation of the liver and can be caused by either infection or toxicity. The majority of cases are caused by viral infections, although occasionally it is caused by parasites. In addition, drugs and alcohol can cause hepatitis, as do hundreds of prescription drugs. As of yet, science has not found a cure for hepatitis. Oil of oregano taken internally, as well as crushed oregano, work very well in killing the infections that cause hepatitis. But in extreme cases, you need to consider all of your options, including oil of oregano, nutritional supplementation, and conventional treatments.

Impetigo: Impetigo is an infection of the skin, which usually appears on the face and is caused by staph or strep. It can spread from one area of the skin to another merely by scratching and then touching another area of the skin. It appears as a red sore that quickly erupts and oozes into a yellowish brown crust. Oil of oregano applied directly to lesions quickly kills staph and strep, so a disciplined regimen will help a lot.

Irritable Bowel Syndrome: "Diseases of the colon are an utter plague of modern humanity, and they are exclusively due to errant diet," says Dr. Ingram. "Parasitic infection is a common cause of irritable bowel syndrome." The crushed oregano is ideal for colonic disorders. It is rich in fiber and minerals like zinc and potassium among others, which aid digestion. Calcium and magnesium from crushed oregano are particularly helpful in relieving cramping. Used in partnership with another herb, *Rhus coriaria*, the contribution to colon health cannot be—nor should be—ignored. Oil of oregano taken internally or added to an enema can be especially helpful.

Laryngitis: Laryngitis occurs when one or both of your vocal cords don't open or close properly. This can be due to viral infection, neck or head injury, thyroid surgery, or tumors of the neck, lungs, and chest. If it is viral, which is generally the case, oil of oregano will kill the virus quickly; but if it does not, see your primary health care provider immediately.

Leukoplakia: Leukoplakia is a common disease of the mouth and is manifested as thick white spots on the mucus membranes and the tongue. Researchers have identified both *Candida albicans* and human papillomavirus, the virus that causes genital warts and cervical cancer, in leukoplakic patches. Again, due to oil of oregano's antiviral properties, a diluted mouthwash may easily handle this infection.

Lichen planus: Lichen planus is a common inflammatory disease of the skin, presenting itself as an itchy, noninfectious rash. A number of infections, mainly hepatitis C virus, are thought to be the cause of *Lichen planus*. Due to oil of oregano's antiviral properties, it may easily handle this infection.

Mastoiditis: Mastoiditis is an infection of the mastoid bone of the skull and is usually a consequence of an ear infection. Once the infection has spread from the ear to the mastoid bone, it fills with infected materials and its honeycomb-like structure may disintegrate. It is important to contact your health care professional immediately if you experience symptoms such as earache, pain behind the ear, redness of the ear and behind the ear, fever, headache, and drainage from the ear. Taken internally, oil of oregano because of its antiviral qualities will kill the infection quickly and should be used before an ear infection progresses to mastoiditis. In other words, don't wait so long that drastic measures have to be taken in order to correct the problem.

Nasal Polyps: Nasal polyps are noncancerous growths in the nasal passages and sinuses. While some nasal polyps are due to infectio and/or allergies, others appear with little to no apparent reason. If you have chronic inflammation of the tissues of the nose and sinuses due to airborne or food allergies you are at a higher risk for nasal polyps than someone with a completely healthy sinus and nasal system. If the cause is due to infection, then oil of oregano will kill the infection. Any other cause should mean a trip to your primary-care physician.

Peptic Ulcer: Folklore held that ulcers were caused by stress and unbalanced amounts of acid in the stomach—anything but what the cause actually was. Researchers in the 1980s found that ulcers were infected with large amounts of a microbe called *Helicobacter pylori*. A few drops of oil of oregano taken internally are highly effective against *Helicobacter pylori*.

Pneumonia: Pneumonia is a very serious infection. Among the elderly in the United States, it is one of the leading causes of death. Pneumonia is an infection of the lung tissue. Viruses, fungi, or bacteria can cause the problem, and in fewer instances, parasites. Whatever the reason, unlike the limited powers of antibiotics, oil of oregano can wipe out the cause quickly and efficiently. Use it the same way as you would for bronchitis.

Psoriasis: According to the American Academy of Dermatology, psoriasis is a chronic, genetic, noncontagious disorder that can affect any part of the body, including the nails and scalp. Physicians believe there is no known cure for psoriasis. But, scientists recently discovered that it is usually caused by a fungal or bacterial infection. Hormonal irregularities like hypothyroidism or adrenal disorders are also connected to psoriasis. Because the organism is not only on the skin, but also in the intestinal tract, treatment must be aimed both internally and externally. A low-sugar or sugar-free diet hastens the treatment. Avoid sugary and starchy foods and eat low-sugar fruits and vegetables. This is a long, extended treatment. According to experts, you should eat primarily meat, fish, eggs, milk products, and vegetables for the first ninety days. Add to this oil of oregano and crushed oregano. The fungal infections that produce psoriasis are virulent and do not give up easily. That's why it is important to stick to the treatment.

Pyorrhea: Pyorrhea is an advanced stage of periodontal disease in which the bone supporting the teeth begins to erode as a result of infection. It causes bad breath, with bleeding and often swollen painful gums. Again, creating a mouthwash of oil of oregano of a few drops of oil in a glass of water or using a drop of oil on your toothbrush can help you maintain excellent dental health.

Rhinitis: Rhinitis is inflammation of the mucus membranes of the nose. There are two types of rhinitis. One type is called allergic rhinitis, which is caused by allergies to foods, common outdoor allergies, molds, or dust. Nonallergic rhinitis is triggered by strong smells, pollution, airborne particulate matter, smoke, or irritants. Whatever the cause, studies have shown that a drop of oil of oregano in a glass of water will provide relief for these symptoms.

Ringworm: This itchy infection is caused by a fungus called tinea. This fungus thrives on a protein in the skin known as keratin. So basically, tinea lives on keratin and the dead skin cells we shed every day. Oregano is extremely effective against this fungus. If you use oil of oregano consistently (apply it directly to the affected area), you should be able to completely kill the fungus within a week or so.

Rosacea: Rosacea is a type of skin rash that generally targets the face—more specifically the nose. Rosacea directly attacks the sebaceous glands, leading to inflammation, redness, and infection. According to studies it appears that the lesions caused by rosacea are infected by parasites. Of course, oil of oregano can handle them.

Scabies: Scabies is an infection of the skin caused by the parasite, *Sarcoptes scabiei*. It is spread primarily through sexual contact but can also be spread through poor hygiene. When the mite gets on your skin, it digs in and starts eating. You will eventually feel severe itching and develop a rash. Scabies can spread to every portion of the skin and you must spread a light film of oil of oregano over the entire body, much in the way the CDC recommends its medication be used. You must soak all potentially exposed clothing, bedding, and other exposed objects in a solution of hot water and two drops of oil to one gallon of hot water. Experts recommend letting all the items soak over night before washing them.

Sinusitis: Sinusitis is characterized by inflammation in the sinus cavities and may be caused by several factors including allergies to pollen or food and bacterial or fungal infection. Researchers at The Mayo Clinic recently found that sinusitis is actually caused by mold infestations—not a pleasant thought. Whatever the source, sinusitis can be excruciatingly painful with waves of pain that feel like you skull is cracking open. It can be stopped before it gets to this point. A few drops of oil of oregano diluted in juice or water will help greatly in this situation.

Sore Throat: Sore throat is caused by bacteria, viruses, or yeast. When a person complains about a sore throat, he or she may be prescribed an antibiotic (if a culture identifies the culprit as bacterial). If it's viral or a yeast, antibiotics will do absolutely nothing—except make those microbes stronger! The beauty of oil of oregano is that it will can kill all three. Try gargling with a weak solution of a few drops of the oil in warm salt water.

Thrush: Thrush is a yeast infection in the mouth. See coated tongue.

Toenail Fungus/Athlete's Foot: Athlete's foot and toenail fungus are caused by a fungus known as dermatophytes. It is an organism that lives off the dead cells sluffed off by our skin every day. It essentially survives on a protein known as keratin, as well as the sugars that are a part our skin, nails, and hair. Once the fungus has gained a foothold it is difficult to eradicate. It can be picked up in public showers, gyms, hotel bathrooms—anywhere public—and then it latches onto your feet. Once it becomes firmly entrenched into the tissues of the skin it does not let go easily.

Fortunately, oil of oregano is able to kill the fungus. However, it is not an easy thing and may take a prolonged treatment. Soak your feet in a warm dilution of several drops of oil or apply the oil directly to affected areas. Keep using the oil as long as you notice improvement until it is completely gone.

Tonsillitis: Tonsillitis is an inflammation of the tonsils, small organs located on either side of the entrance to the throat. The inflammation is usually caused by bacteria, usually streptococcus, but may also be caused by a viral infection. Either way, oil of oregano can handle the situation. Take the oil internally or use in a warm salt water gargle.

Toothache: Toothache is a result of infection. With a milder toothache, there may be a calcium deficiency. So evaluate the severity of your pain, see your dentist, and then apply oil of oregano directly to your tooth for the best results.

Tooth Abscess: A tooth abscess, caused by the presence of harmful bacteria, usually causes severe toothache, a bitter taste, and bad breath. In the extreme, abscesses can cause fever, shivers, and general aches and pains, as well as swelling in the upper and lower jaw and the glands in the neck. If this occurs, get to your doctor immediately. Before it progresses to that stage, apply oil of oregano to combat it.

Ulcerative Colitis: Ulcerative colitis is a disease that causes inflammation and sores, called ulcers, in the lining of the large intestine. The inflammation usually occurs in the rectum and lower part of the colon, but it may affect the entire colon. It rarely affects the small intestine, except for the end section, called the terminal ileum. Ulcerative colitis may also be called colitis or proctitis. Because of oil of oregano's anti-inflammatory properties, along with the healing properties of ice cold aloe juice, it works wonders with colitis.

Warts: Warts are caused by an organism called papillomavirus. Oil of oregano, placed directly on the wart, will aid in the removal of the wart. Clinical studies are still limited in this area, but current results are promising.

Wounds: Oil of oregano is stronger than any other antiseptic you can find, in stores or by prescription. While some will kill microbes, they will also kill human cells. Some prescriptions can cause extensive tissue damage, and some are just plain toxic. Oil of oregano (the P73 variety) is not toxic, does not cause damage to human tissue or become carcinogenic, and it aids in the healing process by keeping the wound free of infection so the body can do what it does best in a balanced circumstance: heal itself. You cannot find a more powerful natural antiseptic.

There are many other health situations where oil of oregano has proven to be beneficial. They include arthritis, sprains, torn or pulled muscles, tendonitis, bursitis, neuritis, back strain, headache, gout, jock itch, cystitis, kidney infection, genital warts, and infected hangnails, to name a few.

So, clearly, oil of oregano does a tremendous amount of healing in many areas—bacterial, fungal, viral, parasitic as well as various organisms.

Various Uses

The uses of oil of oregano, crushed oregano, and juiced oregano are wide and varied. Each aspect has been thoroughly studied and the results published on **www.pubmed.com**, the premier source of medical studies conducted worldwide.

Antibiotic Uses

In a study conducted by I. Dadalioglu and G.A. Evrendilek (Mustafa Kernal University), it was found that carvacrol, one of the primary ingredients in oregano oil, was almost a full 8 percent more effective than the other essential oils in its antibacterial effects. With a 68.23 percent success rate of destroying bacteria, carvacrol led the group.[6]

Oil of oregano was proven in multiple studies to be effective against the following bacterial infections:

actinomycosis	klebsiella
camphylobacter	listeria
cellulitis	Lyme disease
chlamydia	meningitis
cholera	pseudomonas
diphtheria	salmonella
E. coli	shigella
enterobacter	staph
gonorrhea	strep
influenza	tuberculosis

Antifungal Uses

Oil of oregano has been shown to destroy all kinds of fungi. Upon contact, it destroys a wide variety of fungi and yeasts, no matter where they reside. Internally or externally, it has been shown to be remarkably efficient and timely in the dispatch of these nasty little creatures.

In the 1940s and 50s, when nuclear testing was done without discretion, the only form of life that survived contact with nuclear blasts was candida (yeast). But, it didn't survive contact with oil of oregano. When placed in a petri dish with the oregano, it died on contact.

Other fungi oil of oregano has been effective against include:

aspergillus (aspergillosis)   cryptococcal infection
athlete's foot   histoplasmosis
blastomycosis   nocardiosis
Candida albicans   ringworm
coccidiomycosis

Viral Uses

Antibiotics have no effect on viruses, period. Yet Americans rush to the doctor at the first sign of illness and according to some reports, doctors prescribe antibiotics out of fear of malpractice suits or because of the patient's demands. And yet, antibiotics may only make viruses stronger. Viruses actually feed off portions of the antibiotic and change their genetic code.

Numerous studies have been conducted on the effects of oil of oregano on certain viruses. They have found it may be of help with the following:

chicken pox   herpes
cold   measles
cold sores   mumps
croup   pneumonia
encephalitis   shingles
flu   warts
hantavirus   West Nile virus

Antiparasitic Uses

Parasites are a part of everyday life. In some reports, over 80 percent of Americans have some form of parasite wreaking havoc in their bodies. A host of physical ills and ailments can be attributed to parasites residing within the human body. Parasites, such as worms, amoebas, protozoans, and indeed all species of parasites, appear to fall victim to oil of oregano. Other parasites oregano oil has been proven effective against include:

amoebic dysentery   malaria
balantidiasis   pinworm
cryptosporidium   roundworm (aseariasis)

echinococcus (dog tapeworm) shistosomiasis
filariasis   sleeping sickness
giardiasis   tapeworms
hookworm   toxoplasmosis
intestinal flukes   trichomonas
lung flukes

Organisms Destroyed by Oil of Oregano

A number of extremely powerful organisms have met their demise after exposure to oil of oregano. The number of studies conducted on these organisms are fascinating and can be found, along with all the others at **www.pubmed.com**. The following are the organisms destroyed by oil of oregano in the study:

Aspergillus flavus   *Pseudomonas aeruginosa*
Aspergillus parasiticus   *Salmonella typhi*
Aspergillus niger   *Shigella sonnei*
Bacillus subtilis   *Staphylococcus aureus*
Campylobacter jejuni   *Staphylococcus pre*
Candida albicans   *Trichophyton concentricum*
Escherichia coli   *Trichophyton mentagrophtes*
Giardia lamblia   *Trichophyton rubrum*
Helicobacter pylori

Folk Medicine and Oil of Oregano

For nearly five thousand years, oil of oregano has been used as both a savory and a healing herb. While the medical and scientific worlds have finally caught up to folk medicine, traditional remedies are still used to this very day. The Greeks were among the first to begin using oregano oil medicinally, and it has spread throughout the world since that time. The mountainsides of Greece contain fields of oregano, which scent the air with the delicious aroma unique to that herb. Ancient Greeks held the plant in such high esteem that they claimed it was created by the goddess, Aphrodite, as a symbol of happiness. Bridal couples were crowned with garlands of oregano and the plants were placed on tombs to give departed loved ones peace. Turkey, Tibet, Egypt, and various parts of Europe all used oregano as a medicine.

Extensive research has shown the following ailments have long been treated by oil of oregano, crushed oregano, or juiced oregano:

- Ancient Egyptians used it as an emollient and a preservative.
- Ancient Greeks used it to retard spoilage of food as well as for its numerous healing properties. Hippocrates, in the 5th century B.C., prescribed oregano for various diseases, including stomach pain and respiratory diseases. (See Resources at then end of the booklet.)
- In 3,000 BC, ancient Babylonians spoke of oregano as a certain cure for lung and cardiac disease.
- In the 1600s, *Salmons Herbal* identified oregano as the solution for chest, menstrual, uterine, lung, and digestive complaints. *Herbal* went on to detail the usefulness of oregano for diarrhea, asthma, colds, infection of the female sexual organs, uterine tumors, and liver problems. In the 1700s, Gerard, a British herbalist, identified oregano as the complete cure for digestive issues and colds.[15]
- Traditional Chinese doctors have used oregano for centuries to treat fever, vomiting, diarrhea, jaundice, and itchy skin.
- It was used extensively for respiratory problems like coughs, colds, flus, ear aches, and bronchitis.
- Oregano was used for painful menstruation.
- It is used for rheumatoid arthritis.
- It was often recommended for urinary tract infections.
- It is a favorite folk remedy for irritable bowel, diarrhea, constipation, digestive disturbances, bloating, and gas.
- Swollen glands and lack of perspiration received the oregano treatment.
- Oregano was often used as an anti-inflammatory.
- Some suggested it lowered risk of cancer, heart disease, and stroke (this was due to the now proven identification of oregano as a powerful antioxidant).
- It was used for acne.
- Because of its antivenom properties, oregano was used as a

remedy for insect or snake bites.
- Muscle pain received the recommendation of oregano.
- They used it as an antidote.
- Loss of strength received the treatment of the common remedy.
- Oregano was used to reduce fevers.
- Oregano tea helps to relieve an unsettled stomach.
- It eases and soothes a sunburn.

The number of health issues medicinal oregano addresses, both scientifically and in legend, are quite large in number. And, as mentioned previously, hundreds of thousands, if not millions, of people worldwide still cling to the traditions of their forefathers in the use of oregano as the answer to a multitude of health ailments.

Nutritional Value of Oregano

"Wild oregano is a veritable natural treasure trove, containing a density of minerals that would rival, in fact, supersede, any food. The minerals it contains are perhaps too numerous to mention, however, the major ones include calcium, magnesium, iron, phosphorus, copper, zinc, boron, potassium, and manganese. Overall, its density of minerals makes it one of the riches plant sources of trace minerals known."[2]

The minerals located within the oregano plant are more easily absorbed than any other source.

Calcium: 1600 mg per 100 grams. (Richer in calcium than cheese, dark green vegetables, salmon, sardines, and milk.) Calcium is needed for so many elements in the body. Strong bones and teeth, healthy gums, regular heartbeat, healthy heart, blood pressure, cholesterol levels, proper cell membrane permeability, neuromuscular activity, healthy skin, and prevention of pre-eclampsia during pregnancy.[13]

Iron: 50 mg per 100 grams. (Listed as one of the top eight sources of iron.) One of iron's most important functions is the production of hemoglobin and myoglobin as well as the oxygenation of red blood cells. It aids in a healthy immune system, energy production and growth.[13]

Magnesium: 280 mg per 100 grams. (Richer in magnesium than cashews, peanuts, molasses, whole grains, beet greens, and spinach.) Magnesium is vital as a catalyst in enzyme activity, preventing calcification of the soft tissues,and protecting arterial linings from stress.[13]

Zinc: 4 mg per 100 grams. (Richer in zinc than sardines, salmon, cheese, peanut butter, and whole grains.) Zinc is important for the health of the prostate gland, growth of the reproductive organs, healthy immune system, healing of wounds, and acuity of taste and smell.[13]

Copper: 1 mg per 100 grams. Copper aids in the formation of bone, hemoglobin, and red blood cells; the healing process; energy production; hair and skin coloring; taste sensitivity; in maintaining healthy nerves and joints.[13]

Potassium: 1700 mg per 100 grams. (Richer in potassium than orange juice, bananas, apricots, dates, and dark, leafy green vegetables.) Potassium is necessary for a healthy nervous system and a regular heartbeat. It aids in maintaining healthy blood pressure and in transmitting electro-chemical impulses. In addition, it regulates the transfer of nutrients through cell membranes.[13]

As far as vitamins are concerned . . .

Niacin: 6 mg per 100 grams. (Equal to the niacin content of beef, commercial rice, and whole wheat.) Niacin, a part of the vitamin B3, is critical for proper circulation and healthy skins; the nervous system's functions; the metabolism of carbohydrates, fats, and proteins; and the production of hydrochloric acid for the digestive system.[13]

Other vitamins found in oregano include beta-carotene, vitamin C, vitamin K, riboflavin, and thiamine. Oregano is a rich source of bioflavonoids. It is also known as a powerful antioxidant. French researchers measured the ability of spices within the mint family to halt free-radical production. "They noted that oregano possesses 'significant antioxidant activities' and this is largely due to its content of two antioxidant chemicals: rosmarinic and hydroxycinnamic acids."[2]

When tested against other herbs and fruits, previously shown to be high in antioxidants, oregano still reigned supreme.

Cautions

- Oil of oregano may reduce the absorption of iron in your blood. Be certain to use the oil a minimum of two hours before or after taking your vitamin or iron supplements.
- Do not use while pregnant or nursing.
- Oregano is a spice, and allergies to spices are relatively common. Take a single drop of the oregano oil, dilute it with olive or coconut oil, and rub it lightly into your skin. Wait and see if there is any reaction, perhaps several hours, if nothing occurs you are probably pretty safe. If you have a sensitivity to mints, you may be more susceptible to oil of oregano.
- While some doctors say long-term use of the herb is fine, others say it is not and is potentially damaging to the liver and kidneys. This is why the type of oregano used is so critical. The P73 blend of oregano is high in carvacrol, the useful element in oregano, and low in thymol, the harmful element in oregano. Other varieties of oregano are extremely high in thymol. "Only small to moderate amounts of such herbal oils have been deemed safe, and only those that are listed on the FDA's GRAS (Generally Regarded as Safe) list should be consumed. Oil of oregano, of the P73 variety, is one such oil.
- Wild medicinal oregano, the P73 variety, is a very powerful herb and a small amount will do amazing things. Greek researchers in 1995 at the University of Thessonoliki found that a 1 to 4,000 dilution of fresh wild oil of oregano sterilized septic water. Don't go overboard on dosing yourself with oregano. Use caution, common sense and obtain the advice of a naturopath or naturalist familiar with the properties, strengths, and uses of oil of oregano.
- Constipation can occur if excess amounts of oil of oregano are used. This generally does not occur if crushed oregano is used instead of oil of oregano.
- There can be a temporary rise in blood pressure. All spices can cause this occurrence, and yet, interestingly enough, prolonged

exposure normalizes blood pressure.

- If you are on heart medication or multiple medications for any reason, see your health care professional before taking oregano in any of its medicinal forms. The reason for caution is that oregano is a positive ionotrope that strengthens the pumping of the heart.

- Medicinal oregano has strong anti-bacterial properties. If taken for prolonged amounts of time, much like raw garlic, it can kill the good bacteria that reside in the body. If this occurs, the imbalance allows for the growth of *Candida albicans*, which creates a whole new set of problems. So take good bacteria that can be purchased at your local health food store, if needed.

Conclusion

Medicinal oil of oregano is a powerful herb that grows wild on the mountainsides of Greece. At its freshest and most powerful, it will even cause your tongue to go numb. A number of medical studies have proven its effectiveness in a plethora of situations. It behooves each of us to learn more and keep this herb, both crushed and in oil form, in our medicine cabinets.

Again, caution should be taken to insure the oregano has high levels of carvacrol and low levels of thymol. Thymol can be very toxic in high levels. All the testing has proven the P73 version of oregano is the most medicinally strong with the largest amount of the health benefits.

Resources

1. Hortus Third: A Concise Dictionary of Plants Cultivated in the United States and Canada. Wiley/Cornell University, November 1976
2. The Cure is in the Cupboard: How to Use Oregano for Better Health. Dr. Cass Ingram, Knowledge House Publishers, January 1997
3. The Practice of Aromatherapy: A Classic Compendium of Plant Medicines and Their Healing Properties. Jean Valnet and Robert Tisserand, Healing Art Press, December 1990
4. The Wild Oregano Oil Miracle. Dr. Zoltan P. Rona, MD, MSc, http://www.thewolfeclinic.com/oregano.html
5. Journal Applied Microbiology, Volume 86, June 1999
6. Chemical compositions and antibacterial effects of essential oils of Turkish oregano (*Origanum minutiflorum*), Bay Laurel (*Laurus nobilis*), Spanish Lavender (*Lavandula stoechas L.*), and Fennel (*Foeniculum vulgare*) on Common Foodborne Pathogens. Dadalioglu I, Evrendilek GA. Department of Food Engineering, Faculty of Agriculture, Tayfur Sokmen Campus, Mustafa Kemal University, 31034 Alahan, Hatay, Turkey.
7. Antifungal activities of selected aromatic plants growing wild in Greece. Sokovic M, Tzakou O, Pitarokili D, Couladis, M. Department of Plant Physiology, Institute for Biological Research, Belgarde, Yugoslavia. 2002 Oct;46(5):317-20
8. Experimental Study on the Antibacterial Effect of Oraganim Volatile Oil on Dysentary Bacilli in vivo and in vitro. Liao F, Yang Z, Xu H, Gao Q. Department of Microbiology, Tongji Medical College, Huazhong University of Science and Technology, Wuhan 430030, China. 2004;24(4):400-3
9. Antibacterial activities of naturally occurring compounds against antibiotic-resistant *Bacillus cereus* vegetative cells and spores, *Escherichia coli*, and *Staphylococcus aureus*. Friedman M, Buick R, Elliott CT. Western Regional Research Center, Agricultural Research Service, US Department of Agriculture, Albany, California 94710 United States, mfried@pw.usda.gov, 2004 Aug ;67(8):1774-8.
10. Performance of rabbits and oxidative stability of muscle tissues as affected by dietary supplementation with oregano essential oil. Botsoglou NA, Florou-Paneri P, Christaki E, Giannenas I, Spais AB. Laboratory of Animal Nutrition, Faculty of Veterinary Medicine, Aristotle University, Thessaloniki, Greece, bots@veg.auth.gr, 2004 Jun:58(3):209-18.
11. In vitro antioxidant, antimicrobial, and antiviral activities of the essential oil and various extracts from herbal parts and callus cultures of *Origanum acutidens*. Sokmen M, Serkedjieva J, Daferera D, Gulluce M, Polissiou M, Tepe B, Akpulat HA, Sahin F, Sokmen A. Department of

Chemistry, Faculty of Art and Science, Cumhuriyet University, 58 140 Sivas, Turkey. askomen@cumhuriyet.edu.tr, 2004 Jun2;52(11):3309-12.

12. Inhibition of enteric parasites by emulsified oil of oregano in vivo. Force M, Sparks WS, Ronzio RA. Health Explorations Trust, Scottsdale, AZ United States (M.F.) and Biotics Research Corporation, P.O. Box 36888, Houston, Texas, 77236 United States. 2000 May:14(3):213-4.

13. Prescription for Nutritional Healing, Balch, James F. (M.D.), Blach, Phyllis A. (C.N.C.) 1933, 1997, Avery Publishing Group. pp 15, 22-7.

14. Botanical Antibiotics—Oregano Offers Alternative for Fungal, Bacterial Infections. Gulland, Janet: 15 April, 2002, Holistic Primary Care, Vol. 3, No. 1. pp. 1, 12,

15. Wild Oregano Oil: Ancient Remedy. Modern Researcy by Dr. Cass Ingram, D.O., HSR Magazine, 16 January, 2001.

16. Babylonians, Minnesota State University ! Mankato Emuseum, Mankato, Minnesota, United States, Gappa, Andrew, 2003, http://www.mnsu.edu/emuseum/cultural/oldworld/middle_east/babylo-nians.html

17. Hippocrates, University of Virginia, Charlottesville, Virginia, http://www.med.virginia.edu/hslibrary/historical/antiqua/texto.htm

18. Mayo Clinic website, Medline website, National Library of Medicine website and National Institute of Health Web site.

Check out these other top-selling Woodland Health Series booklets:

Ask for them by name or ISBN at your neighborhood bookstore or health-food store. Or call Woodland for the store nearest you.

Açaí Berry	978-1-58054-472-6
Bee Pollen, 2nd Ed.	978-1-58054-429-0
Brain Nutrients, 2nd Ed.	978-1-58054-430-6
Candida Albicans, 2nd Ed.	978-1-58054-432-0
Chelation Therapy, 2nd Ed.	978-1-58054-431-3
Chinese Red Yeast Rice, 2nd Ed.	978-1-58054-434-4
Coconut Oil	978-1-58054-464-1
CoQ10 (All new!)	978-1-58054-456-8
Cranberry	978-1-58054-461-0
CLA, 2nd Ed.	978-1-58054-433-7
Colon Health, 2nd Ed.	978-1-58054-435-1
Digestive Enzymes, 2nd Ed.	978-1-58054-436-8
Essential Fatty Acids, 2nd Ed.	978-1-58054-437-5
Flaxseed Oil, 2nd Ed.	978-1-58054-438-2
Hyaluronic Acid	978-1-58054-458-0
Influenza, Epidemics, Bird Flu	978-1-58054-425-2
Ginkgo Biloba, 2nd Ed.	978-1-58054-484-9
Ginseng (All new!)	978-1-58054-483-2
Glucosamine Chondroitin, 2nd Ed.	978-1-58054-439-9
Goji	978-1-58054-473-3
Grapefruit Seed Extract, 2nd Ed.	978-1-58054-446-7
Green Tea, 2nd Ed.	978-1-58054-440-5
Hoodia, 2nd Ed.	978-1-58054-448-1

Managing Acid Reflux, 2nd Ed.	978-1-58054-444-3
Mangosteen	978-1-58054-470-2
Miracle Sugars, 2nd Ed.	978-1-58054-449-8
Nattokinase	978-1-58054-474-0
Natural Guide to Alzheimers	978-1-58054-423-8
Natural Guide to Back Pain	978-1-58054-457-3
Natural Guide to Energy Enhancement	978-1-58054-414-6
Natural Guide to Fertility	978-1-58054-466-5
Natural Guide to Headaches	978-1-58054-443-6
Natural Guide to HPV	978-1-58054-463-4
Natural Guide to Managing Pre-Diabetes	978-1-58054-465-8
Natural Guide to Liver Health	978-1-58054-397-2
Olive Leaf Extract, 2nd Edition	978-1-58054-441-2
Stevia, 2nd Edition	978-1-58054-476-4
Stress, 2nd Edition	978-1-58054-477-1
Supplements for Fibromyalgia, 2nd Ed.	978-1-58054-442-9
Xylitol	978-1-58054-139-8

Can't find a title you're looking for? Woodland has more than 150 different Woodland Health Series booklets and 60+ full-length books on health and wellness. Ask someone at the store where you got this booklet for more information.

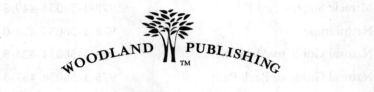